How To Get The Most From Acupuncture Treatments

289 Great Acupuncture Tips To Keep You Healthy And Happy

ADAM COLTON

Published by BizMove
www.bizmove.com

Disclaimer

ISBN: 1979334420
ISBN- 978-1979334426

289 Great Acupuncture Tips To Keep You Healthy And Happy

Acupuncture has been practiced in China and other Asian countries for thousands of years. Acupuncture involves stimulating specific points on the body. This is most often done by inserting thin needles through the skin, to cause a change in the physical functions of the body.

Acupuncture is a healing art that uses your body's own abilities to heal itself. It does not add anything foreign to your body and takes nothing away. It is an ancient art and entirely natural. If you want to learn about acupuncture, read the tips presented here. Let acupuncture work for you.

1. It is important to let your acupuncturist know about the vitamins or medications you are taking before the beginning of your treatment. Some pills can affect your system and counteract the effects of an acupuncture session. You might have to stop taking your medication or vitamins for a while if you want to get good results from acupuncture.

2. Think ahead before you schedule your next acupuncture appointment. Its best that you don't have a session right before or right after you do

something strenuous. If you usually workout on Wednesdays, make your appointment on a Thursday. If you're expecting to have a stressful couple of days, schedule your appointment for the following week. Acupuncture works best when you're truly able to relax.

3. Make sure your acupuncturist received licensure through the State Health Department. You do not want to end up with an under-qualified practitioner. You can be sure that they know what they're doing.

4. If you'd like to get more out of your acupuncture sessions, start cleansing. A good cleanse will free your body of toxins, which means acupuncture will be more effective. During this time, you may also want to detox from substances like alcohol. Ask your acupuncturist to recommend a good detox diet.

5. Be sure to wear layered, loose, comfortable clothing to your acupuncture sessions. You have to ensure your practitioner is able to reach what they have to reach. Taking off clothing is a choice, but it is simpler if you have a wardrobe that is flexible.

6. Inquire about the length of each session. If you have several conditions to treat it may lengthen the session, but it usually lasts around 30 minutes. Don't make plans for an appointment immediately following acupuncture treatment. It is best to simply rest and relax.

7. Never fight an acupuncture treatment during the middle of it. You've made the decision to get this treatment, hopefully reading up prior to the appointment. If you start tensing up or responding poorly (both physically and verbally), you can be sure that the session won't give you the best results.

8. Do not go to your acupuncture appointment hungry or full. Make sure to have a healthy snack about an hour before your appointment. Do not go with an empty stomach or after a large meal. Being to full or hungry way makes it much more difficult to relax during your acupuncture appointment.

9. As you would with many other services, schedule a consultation with any prospective acupuncturists. These generally last 10-15 minutes, but they can give you an idea of whether or not they are right for you. Ask them any questions that you have, talk about their

experience and education, express any concerns, and pay attention to how they make you feel in their office. If you ever feel uncomfortable, try someone else.

10. Ask your acupuncturist if there are certain herbs you should consume in between sessions. Remember, this is a holistic practice. There are many different things to it compared to Western medicine. Herbs are a big part of it. They can help relax your body and remove any sort of pain left over from your session.

11. When choosing an acupuncturist, ask your friends and relatives for a recommendation. Acupuncture has become so popular that it will not be hard for you to find someone who has tried it. Getting a recommendation from someone you know is the best way to find an acupuncturist who is experienced and reliable.

12. Discuss acupuncture with any friends or relatives who have received this type of treatment. Find out what they experienced. Ask how it has affected their well-being. If you take the time to learn a lot prior to going to a session, acupuncture won't make you feel so stressed. Be open to exploring the subject.

13. Sometimes acupuncture can leave you feeling sore, particularly on your feet and hands. Generally, the soreness will go away in a day's time, although you may experience some issues for up to a week later. Simply try to stay off your feet as much as possible, and allow your hands to rest as well.

14. It's ok to nap a bit during your session. Falling asleep is ok. Meditating is even better, but it can be tough to not let tiredness overtake you when you are this relaxed for up to an hour. Meditating or sleeping, though, are really where you should draw the line. No reading or stressing over business or personal problems.

15. As you choose between the varieties of acupuncturist, you need to know what each offers. One option is a medical doctor who has had one to two hundred hours of training in acupuncture. They need to be an American Academy of Medical Acupuncture member for you to be sure they know what they're doing.

16. If you wear a pacemaker, you should be careful. You may find that your acupuncture treatment combines the use of needles and electrical pulses. This is usually not a problem. But, if you are someone with a pacemaker, such pulses can

interfere with its operation. If you have one, make sure that your acupuncturist knows about it before your treatment begins.

17. Acupuncture can relieve stress on the long term. If you have a hard time coping with your stressful lifestyle, consider meeting with your acupuncturist a couple times a month. You will notice an improvement on the long term but keep in mind that you will also have to make some changes to your lifestyle.

18. Keep in mind that it may take some time for you to feel the full benefits from your acupuncture treatments. It may take more than one or two visits to find relief from pain or improvement in your conditions. Make sure you are ready to commit to the full program recommended.

19. Familiarize yourself with acupuncture before your first session. Needles will play a major role in the treatment. They're necessary for the process. If they usually make you nervous, you should try to face this fear head on. If you have to, talk to other people that have done acupuncture in the past and see how their experience went so you can feel at ease.

20. Think ahead before you schedule your next acupuncture appointment. Its best that you don't have a session right before or right after you do something strenuous. If you usually workout on Wednesdays, make your appointment on a Thursday. If you're expecting to have a stressful couple of days, schedule your appointment for the following week. Acupuncture works best when you're truly able to relax.

21. Ask any potential acupuncturist how many years they have been in business. As with most other professions, experience counts for a lot. You also want to find out where they received their education. There is often a big difference in quality if the person trained in the United States versus somewhere else.

22. If you frequently suffer from coughs or colds, ask your acupuncturist to work on Lung 7. This will help you get rid of neck pain, but it will also help strengthen your lungs. When your lungs are in good shape, little bugs won't hit you as hard. This is especially useful during wintertime.

23. It is always best to ask a few questions to the acupuncturists you are interested in before scheduling an appointment. You need to ask if the acupuncturist is certified by the NCCAOM.

The only way to get this certification is to earn a medical degree and do an acupuncture internship.

24. Let your acupuncturist know if you're taking any medicines. That knowledge will help them devise an appropriate treatment plan for you.

25. Avoid having coffee before your treatment. You should abstain for about two hours before an appointment. This restriction is due to the fact that coffee is a stimulant which works in direct opposition to the goals of your acupuncture session. Coffee also makes the acupuncturist's job more difficult because it is harder to get accurate heart rate readings.

26. Watch for practitioners that tell you they have therapies that can cure HIV, cancer, and other serious diseases. Acupuncture does offer relief for many different ailments, but it is not a magical cure. Make sure to see these treatments for exactly what they can do, but do not avoid conventional medicine when dealing with something severe.

27. Don't look at your acupuncture session as a time to pick up a book. Yes, you are laying quietly for up to an hour, but it's your job to relax--even

meditate if you want to--during the session. Your practitioner needs your help in this matter. The more relaxed you are, the better the session will be.

28. Does your work insurance not cover acupuncture? Then, talk to your coworkers about starting a campaign. If your coworkers agree that acupuncture should be covered, get together as a group and contact your human resources department. If you can get enough people to follow you, you might be able to get it added into your benefits.

29. Acupuncture is recognized as an effective treatment for a lot of different ailments and diseases by the medical world. If you are considering having this type of treatment, you might want to check with your insurance company first. Many insurance companies will actually cover the cost of acupuncture treatments.

30. Rest and relax immediately after your treatment. Reduce daily activities and avoid strenuous physical activities. Make sure you get to bed on time so you can get a full night's sleep. A rested body will respond to treatment better than a tired one.

31. Educate yourself on acupuncture before you go for a session. Read up on both Oriental acupuncture and modern practices. You may also want to speak to practitioners. When it comes to acupuncture, many people are skeptical. It'll be easier to avoid that skepticism and trust in your acupuncturist when you know more about its history.

32. You should not drink coffee before an acupuncture treatment. Coffee has stimulation properties and will make it hard for you to relax during your treatment. Your acupuncturist will have a hard time measuring your pulse if you drink coffee. If possible, wait until after your appointment to have some coffee.

33. It is best to receive your acupuncture treatments on a regular basis. Schedule two weekly appointments for your first month and change the frequency of your appointments in function of how efficient they are. If your chronic pain or your stress is mostly gone, a monthly appointment might be enough.

34. If you don't know anyone who has seen an acupuncturist, check online reviews for practitioners in your area. Also contact the Better

Business Bureau and any nearby Chamber of Commerce. They will provide you with any complaints which may have been filed against the practitioners you are considering, so take note.

35. Find out if the acupuncturists you are considering offer other treatments as well. For example, some chiropractors also offer acupuncture, so getting them both done with one doctor may be beneficial. Other practitioners may offer reiki healing, herbal or naturopathic treatments or other Chinese medical treatments, offering you a holistic approach to health.

36. Never visit an acupuncturist who uses the same needles over and over again! If they don't get new needles from out of a sterile sealed pack, ask them where their needles came from. Used needles can be very dangerous and cause you to develop an infection.

37. Avoid over-eating right before your acupuncture appointment. Although you should not go on an empty stomach, as this can lead to feeling dizzy, you can't be too full either. Call and ask for guidance with the receptionist if you're not sure, but don't take any chances by indulging in a big meal a few hours prior to going.

38. Do your research on the acupuncturists in your area. Avoid choosing an acupuncturist who has any unresolved complaints. Check with your local Better Business Bureau and do some online research before choosing an acupuncturist. You're more likely to have a positive experience if you do your research first.

39. Ask your acupuncturist how many years of experience they have. It is important to choose a doctor who has been practicing for at least five years to make sure they know what they are doing. Look for reviews on the Internet and ask your acupuncturist for a few references if you want to learn more about their methods.

40. Did you know that acupuncture can be of assistance to those looking to quit smoking? The actual acupuncture procedure helps people deal with the side effects of nicotine addiction, like irritability, cravings and jitters. It calms the patient down so they are better able to deal with these side effects.

41. Acupuncture can help you get more energy. If you have a hard time with going through your daily tasks and often feel drained, find an acupuncturist. You should explain them your

problems and they will be able to help you thanks to a treatment designed to boost your energy level.

42. If you are interested in acupuncture but cannot afford it, ask your practitioner if they will accept you as a patient on a sliding scale. Many practitioners offer this service, as they realize the health benefits offered by this therapy. Typically, you will pay only what you can afford or agree to a bulk payment for several treatments.

43. If you have an insurance company that doesn't cover acupuncture, try starting a campaign to write them letters. If you have colleagues who wish to undergo acupuncture treatment, recruit them to speak to Human Resources officers. If enough people show interest in acupuncture, an insurance company is more likely to cover it.

44. Acupuncture rarely is painful in any way. The needles used in acupuncture are very thin. You can barely see them with the naked eye. Because of their small size, they often do not hit nerve endings and you will feel no pain. Even when they do hit a nerve, they are so small you barely feel it.

45. Oftentimes after your first acupuncture visit, you will feel some immediate pain relief. This is fairly common. Acupuncture has been practiced for thousands of years and these practitioners know what they are doing. Although acupuncture is not recognized as a medical treatment, for some people it can actually cure their chronic pain.

46. You might be more sensitive than usual after an acupuncture treatment. Do not worry if you experience mood swings or seem to cry very easily. This is a sign that your acupuncture treatment is working well. These symptoms should eventually disappear as you get used to receiving acupuncture treatments regularly.

47. Some patients experience a runny nose or slight flu like symptoms following an acupuncture treatment. In Chinese medicine, it is believed that colds and flus are at the root of many ailments within the body. These symptoms are just the body's way of releasing toxins, and they typically do not last for long. Do your best to keep yourself comfortable during this time, and you will soon return to optimum health.

48. Be prepared to answer questions during your very first acupuncture appointment. A first

appointment can last as much as two hours since your acupuncturist needs to know about your medical history. Make sure to be clear and honest with your acupuncturist to get the best treatment.

49. Get yourself into a relaxed state before beginning your acupuncture treatment. Life is full of tensions, from work assignments to family arguments. Leave those behind when you get on the acupuncture table. The more you're able to relax, the better you'll respond to the treatments given. That's where you want to be.

50. It is important to communicate with your practitioner as they treat you. The needles they use are very thin, so discomfort should be minimal and should amount to nothing more than tingling or aching. If you become uncomfortable at any time, let the practitioner know so that they can alter your treatment as necessary.

51. If a practitioner you are considering reuses their needles, run for the hills! A good acupuncturist uses single use needles which are safely disposed of once done. The rest of the office should be sterilized as necessary. Your practitioner, if

licensed, has to take safety courses to be licensed, so they should know the ropes.

52. Do not ask the acupuncturist how many times you will need to see them before you are cured. Every person is unique and nobody can tell you when you feel better. That is something only you will know. Keep going until you are feeling better and do not feel the need to seek treatment.

53. Consider writing a review for your acupuncturist if you enjoyed a favorable experience. Many people are still unfamiliar with this therapy option, and your input will help instruct others about the positive effects. If you've had a positive experience, share it online or among your friends. This will make you feel good, and you'll be helping your practitioner gain business.

54. It is important to relax before going to an acupuncture treatment. If you are tense, the needles will not be able to get past your clenched muscles. Breathing deeply just before the treatment or listening to some relaxing music should help. If you are having problems with tensed muscles, let your acupuncturist know about this problem.

55. Do not be surprised if you feel a tingling sensation during your acupuncture treatment. Introducing pins in your skin should cause you to experience a sensation known as Qi. A lot of beginners associate this sensation with pain at first but you will soon realize that you are not actually hurting.

56. Acupuncture produces different effects in different people. Some people report that they feel extremely relaxed after a session, while others notice a burst of extra energy. A common benefit reported by most patients is an overall sense of well-being and fitness. These feelings are in addition to achieving the pain relief they were seeking.

57. Keep an open mind. Regardless of what you thought about acupuncture in the past, remember that a large number of patients often report feeling better the day they receive their treatment. Go in to your appointment and maintain an optimistic outlook. You will feel better about everything that is going on if you do.

58. While you may appreciate the work your acupuncturist is doing, don't feel the need to tip. Acupuncturists are similar to medical

professionals like doctors rather than beauticians. These people are health care professionals, and this is a field that normally does not receive tips.

59. Do not just go to one appointment and then stop. Generally, you will experience the best results if you go to several treatments. If you are not dedicated to the process, you are not going to benefit as much from it. Talk to your doctor about what you can realistically expect after the first appointment and then going forward.

60. If you go abroad, avoid going to see an acupuncturist. Acupuncture is very popular in most Asian countries but keep in mind that the acupuncturist do not have the same education as the doctors who treated you in the past. These doctors might not have high hygiene standards or not practice painless acupuncture.

61. Determine if and how your insurance plan covers acupuncture. Some plans cover acupuncture only if you are referred by your regular practitioner for a medical condition. Other plans cover acupuncture visits as wellness visits. Find out if your health insurance covers acupuncture so you can save some cash on the procedure.

62. Understand that acupuncture focus on the entire well being of you as a person. In Western culture, it's often the norm to concentrate on symptoms, what's ailing you immediately. That's not true of acupuncture. It looks at the big picture and tries to help your entire body. It's a major difference in thought.

63. Be sure the acupuncturist doing the procedure on you is experienced and knows what they are doing. Though rare, one wrong move and the needle could pierce through an organ, such as your lungs. Should this occur, you could end up suffering from internal bleeding. You are less likely to have to worry about this if your acupuncturist is experienced.

64. Acupuncture pins are meant to target the chi in the body. Chi refers to your life force energy. There is an energy channel in the body and anytime there is an obstruction or anything that interferes with it, it takes the form of a physical issue in the body like pain. The pins in acupuncture can help redirect or balance the chi in your body.

65. When you schedule your session, mention any vitamins or supplements you've been taking. Your acupuncturist may want you to temporarily

cease taking some of them. While providing your body with extra nutrients is always a good thing, some of the supplements may cause mild side effects when taken on the day of an acupuncture session.

66. Even if you are a skeptic when it comes to acupuncture, do your best to keep an open mind. Scientific studies are ongoing regarding the effectiveness of such treatments, and there is new information being discovered all the time. Keep up to date on current research, discuss your findings with your doctor and consider acupuncture treatments for your health conditions. This just might help you to find the relief you have been looking for.

67. Figure out how long you will be at your appointment before going. It is important to stay relaxed after your treatment, and you will not stay calm if you immediately begin rushing because you are behind in your schedule. Also, learn the length of time that your treatment will take.

68. Eat well after your acupuncture session. Keep in mind that acupuncture helps remove harmful toxins from your body. Don't eat junk food after your acupuncture treatment or you will undo all

the good work that has been done. Therefore, consume lots of fruits and vegetables so you can keep your body and mind healthy.

69. Ask about vitamins, herbal remedies or medicines you may be taking. Your acupuncturist can help you determine if any of these need to be postponed before your treatment. Sometimes you may need to avoid taking them between sessions as well. Consult first and you will know exactly how to increase the benefits.

70. Beware of sticker shock. Call your insurance company before getting any treatments. Not every insurance company covers acupuncture. In fact, quite a few cover no forms of alternative medicine at all. Know if that's the case for you before you step into your sessions. You may not like the bill at the end otherwise.

71. Eat a light meal before your appointment. If you eat too much then you may have trouble reaching the results that the session was supposed to give you. It is not a good idea to go into an acupuncture treatment while you are hungry either. You could end up passing out during the treatment.

72. Remember that acupuncture does not use needles. Many people think that they are being stuck with small needles that hurt, but this isn't the case. Tiny, solid and sterile little pins that are about the thickness of a strand of hair are what are used for acupuncture. Many of them are flexible, and since they aren't hollow, they rarely cause pain.

73. Ask any potential acupuncturist how many years they have been in business. As with most other professions, experience counts for a lot. You also want to find out where they received their education. There is often a big difference in quality if the person trained in the United States versus somewhere else.

74. Make sure you don't see your acupuncturist on an empty stomach. You'll want to eat a full meal about 2 hours before your session. If you go to a session hungry, you may wind up feeling dizzy or lightheaded. You want your sessions to make you feel better, not worse.

75. Keep in mind that the benefits of acupuncture might not be found after one session. Sometimes, it takes time for your body to learn to utilize energy properly and the pressure points used in acupuncture to work correctly. This

might mean that you have to undergo several sessions before seeing the results you are hoping for.

76. Contact your insurance provider before seeking acupuncture treatments. Some plans will cover most or all of the cost of this treatment, but you might need a referral from your general practitioner first. Take the time to make a call to your insurance company first so you are not left with surprise bills after treatment is received.

77. Inquire whether you should do anything before or after your treatment. Your acupuncturist may want you to take certain actions, such as laying down for a while after the treatment, or drinking a full glass of water. Find out before your treatment, so you know what to expect each time.

78. If you are actively looking for a new acupuncturist, it is a very good idea to look for reviews prior to making an appointment. While everyone will not have the same experience, you should see it as a bad sign if you do not find any positive reviews at all.

79. If you are interested in acupuncture but cannot afford it, ask your practitioner if they will accept

you as a patient on a sliding scale. Many practitioners offer this service, as they realize the health benefits offered by this therapy. Typically, you will pay only what you can afford or agree to a bulk payment for several treatments.

80. All acupuncture needles should be labeled for single use only. Make sure this is the case in your acupuncturists office. Ask to see the needles, and make sure they are bagged appropriately and labeled for single use. If this is not the case, you could risk exposure to dangerous diseases.

81. Before accepting treatment, make sure you see the needles being used. All needles for acupuncture must be sterile and marked for one time use. This is an important aspect of your health safety. If you didn't see the needles unwrapped in front of you, ask for a new set.

82. If your acupuncturist has less than ten years of experience, ask for references. While you might be able to find a practitioner who is newer to the field and still very good, you want to make sure to proceed with caution in such a case. An inexperienced practitioner might not know how to treat you properly, and this could put your health in danger.

83. You should not expect too much from your acupuncture treatments. Acupuncture can efficiently relieve pain and stress but it will not help you improve your health. You need to make some changes to your lifestyle if you suffer from chronic pain or often feel stressed. Your acupuncturist can provide you with some useful tips on how to improve your lifestyle.

84. Form an opinion about acupuncture before you get any sessions. For some, acupuncture is bunk. For others, it is a potentially potent treatment for overall health. No, you won't know totally what side of the fence you're on until after your full sessions, but if it's obviously not for you up front, don't go into it at all. Look to other solutions.

85. If you cannot afford an acupuncture treatment, look into going to a community acupuncture session. These sessions take place in large and quiet rooms where several patients are treated at the same time. You will still get a chance to explain your problems and get a customized treatment from a qualified acupuncturist.

86. Don't expect acupuncture overnight miracles. This is not a miracle cure. It's something that will take multiple sessions and a lot of focus to bring

the best results. If you're expecting immediate benefits, acupuncture may not be the right treatment for you. Consult your doctor for other alternatives that might be better fits for you.

87. The best option when choosing a practitioner is to go with a Licensed Acupuncturist. They actually have an Oriental Medicine or Acupuncture degree, proving they have the training to do it right. They have as many as 2,400 hours of education behind them, unlike the one to two hundred physicians or chiropractors have.

88. It is important to relax before going to an acupuncture treatment. If you are tense, the needles will not be able to get past your clenched muscles. Breathing deeply just before the treatment or listening to some relaxing music should help. If you are having problems with tensed muscles, let your acupuncturist know about this problem.

89. Prepare yourself for needles. Acupuncture involves needles and there isn't a way around it. Confront any needle issues you have head on. Try to get yourself prepared for needles before your appointment, otherwise you may feel anxious.

90. When seeking a professional acupuncture practitioner, make sure to solicit recommendations from those you know and also spend some time reading reviews online. By taking these steps, you can ensure that you are spending your time and your money wisely and that you will receive the maximum benefits possible from this sort of treatment.

91. Some people find acupuncture treatments are quite effective for migraine headaches. One very positive aspect of this type of alternative treatment is the lack of any side effects. Even though very fine needles are inserted into the flesh at specific points, most people do not feel any pain at all from the procedure.

92. If you're apprehensive about visiting a chiropractor, fear not! The needles are not nearly as large as the one your physician uses, and most people report hardly feeling them at all. The minor discomfort you may feel from a session of acupuncture will be well worth the total relief you will feel thereafter!

93. Understand that acupuncture focus on the entire well being of you as a person. In Western culture, it's often the norm to concentrate on

symptoms, what's ailing you immediately. That's not true of acupuncture. It looks at the big picture and tries to help your entire body. It's a major difference in thought.

94. Don't wear clothes that are too tight when you have an acupuncture appointment. Loose clothing is a better choice since your acupuncturist needs access to different points. The needles will be easier to place because of the access provided by the loose clothing. There are group acupuncture sessions in which all participants remain fully clothed. Loose clothing is essential in this setting.

95. Do not go to your acupuncture appointment hungry or full. Make sure to have a healthy snack about an hour before your appointment. Do not go with an empty stomach or after a large meal. Being to full or hungry way makes it much more difficult to relax during your acupuncture appointment.

96. If you feel very tired after an acupuncture treatment, you should get some rest. Acupuncture is supposed to give you some energy but you will not get this positive effect if you need some sleep. It is important to get eight hours of sleep a night until your next treatment.

97. Consider looking at specialized acupuncture treatments. Acupuncture, like traditional medicine, is a vast field, so you are bound to find treatments and acupuncturists that specialize in specific areas. For instance, there is acupuncture that specializes in just migraines and headaches or just chronic pain and stress. You might want to find someone that knows specialized treatments for your particulate ailments.

98. Is arthritis, back pain or a bad headache a regular problem for you? Have you tried nearly everything to cease the pain, but not had any results? You may wish to try acupuncture. It's a natural treatment which allows your body to heal itself, which is great for pain relief.

99. Give seasonal acupuncture treatment a try. Seasonal treatments involve aligning your body to the present season changes. The fall and winter seasons are cold; therefore, you are more likely to experience respiratory issues, such as a cold and congestion. That means the lungs should be targeted. Pay attention to what the acupuncturist suggests and consider adding them to your normal routine.

100.   Some patients experience a runny nose or slight flu like symptoms following an acupuncture treatment. In Chinese medicine, it is believed that colds and flus are at the root of many ailments within the body. These symptoms are just the body's way of releasing toxins, and they typically do not last for long. Do your best to keep yourself comfortable during this time, and you will soon return to optimum health.

101.   One of the most important things to remember during your acupuncture treatment is to relax. The procedure will not work as well if you are tense or anxious. Inform your acupuncturist if you feel burning, itching or pain during treatment. If you end up with an itch, you could ruin the whole procedure.

102.   If your acupuncturist has less than ten years of experience, ask for references. While you might be able to find a practitioner who is newer to the field and still very good, you want to make sure to proceed with caution in such a case. An inexperienced practitioner might not know how to treat you properly, and this could put your health in danger.

103.   Ask plenty of questions to your acupuncturist before and after a treatment. You

can learn a lot about acupuncture if you ask your acupuncturist to describe the treatment they are about to administer and talk about the sensations you experienced after the treatment. You will be able to ask for the same treatment again if you know what your acupuncturist did.

104.   In most areas, an acupuncturist has to have a license. Ask to see this as you are interviewing your potential choices. These licenses often call for thousands of hours of training along with being recertified from time to time. Actual medical doctors don't need a licence to practice acupuncture, though.

105.   There is a lot more to acupuncture than the treatments involving needles. This medicinal practice is associated with a philosophy. You should learn more about the philosophy of acupuncture to adopt a healthier lifestyle. There are plenty of meditation exercises, home remedies and other practices you can use to introduce acupuncture in the different aspects of your life.

106.   Acupuncture produces different effects in different people. Some people report that they feel extremely relaxed after a session, while others notice a burst of extra energy. A common

benefit reported by most patients is an overall sense of well-being and fitness. These feelings are in addition to achieving the pain relief they were seeking.

107.   If you are too scared of needles, laser acupuncture is another option. This light therapy applies lasers to the body's pressure points. This doesn't hurt a bit, and it is quite effective.

108.   Increases in energy is among the real benefits of acupuncture. Many clients have reported an increased level of energy for weeks after their sessions. People are usually relaxed immediately after a treatment, but the energy boost soon follows.

109.   Determine if and how your insurance plan covers acupuncture. Some plans cover acupuncture only if you are referred by your regular practitioner for a medical condition. Other plans cover acupuncture visits as wellness visits. Find out if your health insurance covers acupuncture so you can save some cash on the procedure.

110.   Be sure you set aside time to relax prior to your acupuncture appointment and afterwards as well. Your body is going to better respond when

your body is relaxed, and the practitioner can more easily attend to his craft. Lay back and enjoy being treated with one of the most relaxing procedures available.

111.   An acupuncturist might not be a medical doctor, but you should still be sure that they're aware of your medical history. Fill them in on your family's health issues, and make sure they know about any medications you've been taking. The more information they have, the better picture they'll have of your health and the more they'll be able to do to help you.

112.   If you are actively looking for a new acupuncturist, it is a very good idea to look for reviews prior to making an appointment. While everyone will not have the same experience, you should see it as a bad sign if you do not find any positive reviews at all.

113.   Although your life may be busy, it is important to relax after your acupuncture session. This is important to help calm your nerves after the procedure. Try to sleep for at least eight hours after completing a session.

114.   Do some research about the different kinds of acupuncture before you begin looking for an

acupuncture practitioner. American acupuncturists can practice based on traditions from Korea, China or Japan. Always ask about your practitioner's training and exactly what kind of procedures they use. It is also helpful to find out if one branch of acupuncture is more effective than another for your particular condition.

115.   Acupuncture can help you get more energy. If you have a hard time with going through your daily tasks and often feel drained, find an acupuncturist. You should explain them your problems and they will be able to help you thanks to a treatment designed to boost your energy level.

116.   Get a full description of what your treatment will be like. Treatments differ based off of what a person is going through, so don't expect your treatment to mirror what your friend received. Your acupuncturist, though, should be able to describe what to expect as you go through the sessions.

117.   Some people get light headed after a treatment, although not many. Make sure you get up from the table slowly, and always have a snack before you head in for your appointment.

If you notice any light headedness, don't rush to get out of the building. Sit down for a while to see if you feel better.

118.   Check up on the professionalism of your acupuncturist prior to selecting the practitioner. This means doing a little research. Talk to your friends and peers, and do some online research. Make sure there are no obvious red flags that should hold you back from getting involved with their establishment.

119.   Bring along a comfort object. This is especially important during the first few sessions. This will relieve the excess tension that you have during your session. Ask your acupuncturist if you can bring the item with you to your session.

120.   The best option when choosing a practitioner is to go with a Licensed Acupuncturist. They actually have an Oriental Medicine or Acupuncture degree, proving they have the training to do it right. They have as many as 2,400 hours of education behind them, unlike the one to two hundred physicians or chiropractors have.

121.   When you are interviewing your potential practitioners in person, ask them how many

treatments they think it will take to heal you. If you receive an answer, you should cross that acupuncturist off your list. There is no way to know how quickly you will heal, so they should tell you as much.

122.   Acupuncture is a great remedy for digestive issues. In fact, it can help with many natural cycles, including digestion. Speak to your practitioner about diet so you can boost your nutrition and reap maximum benefits from the treatment. Continue your regular appointments until you see improvement in your digestion.

123.   Don't get into your car to visit an acupuncturist without knowing in advance what lies ahead of you. You're going to have to work with needles. It is simply part of the process. If they make you anxious, you need to confront the fear directly. Talk to people who have been through it before and gain confidence from their successes.

124.   You should find out if your acupuncturist is NCCAOM certified before you set an appointment. This national board certifies practitioners that have completed a national exam and full program. It doesn't say anything about whether their sessions are painful or not,

but it does mention their educational level describing how many hours were spent in school and if they did any supervised internships at their school's clinic.

125.   If you have some fear of acupuncture because you think that it is going to hurt, ask your acupuncturist about techniques in painless needling. Ask questions about where he learned that technique and how long he has been practicing it. Only go with practitioners who have had multiple years of experience.

126.   Ask any potential acupuncturist how many years they have been in business. As with most other professions, experience counts for a lot. You also want to find out where they received their education. There is often a big difference in quality if the person trained in the United States versus somewhere else.

127.   Do not expect to leave your first appointment feeling one-hundred percent better. Like many treatments, it will take a few visits before you reach full levels of restoration. Be patient and give the treatment a chance before you call it quits. You will be happy you gave it enough time.

128. Make sure you don't see your acupuncturist on an empty stomach. You'll want to eat a full meal about 2 hours before your session. If you go to a session hungry, you may wind up feeling dizzy or lightheaded. You want your sessions to make you feel better, not worse.

129. You should drink plenty of water before you attend your scheduled acupuncture session. It has been shown that people who are well hydrated respond better to treatments. While you should not consume a lot of food before a session, it is a great idea for you to drink a good amount of water.

130. Inquire about the length of each session. Acupuncture sessions usually last for half an hour, but some sessions take longer. Don't plan anything within an hour of your appointment to give you time to relax.

131. Inquire whether you should do anything before or after your treatment. Your acupuncturist may want you to take certain actions, such as laying down for a while after the treatment, or drinking a full glass of water. Find out before your treatment, so you know what to expect each time.

132.   Some people should not have acupuncture done. For example, pregnant women should avoid it because it can cause premature labor. Those with pacemakers should not have it done because electrical pulses may be applied to the needles, which may stop a pacemaker from functioning properly. Speak with your doctor before having acupuncture done to be sure it is safe for you.

133.   If you're a workout fanatic, you'll no doubt want to exercise on session day. Exercise is okay, however, avoid strenuous exercises. A walk is more acceptable than a rigorous run, in this case. The day of your appointment should be a day of mild stretching, rather than strenuous exercises.

134.   Eat properly following acupuncture sessions. One of the goals of acupuncture is to draw out your toxins. If you indulge in unhealthy foods following your visit, you are adding more toxins to your body. Try eating lots of fresh produce instead.

135.   Some patients experience a runny nose or slight flu like symptoms following an acupuncture treatment. In Chinese medicine, it is believed that colds and flus are at the root of many ailments within the body. These symptoms

are just the body's way of releasing toxins, and they typically do not last for long. Do your best to keep yourself comfortable during this time, and you will soon return to optimum health.

136.   Ask about vitamins, herbal remedies or medicines you may be taking. Your acupuncturist can help you determine if any of these need to be postponed before your treatment. Sometimes you may need to avoid taking them between sessions as well. Consult first and you will know exactly how to increase the benefits.

137.   Study up on acupuncture. You've probably heard of it, and if you have, you know it involves needles. But there is much more to acupuncture, and you should get a better picture of it prior to making any decisions about it. Remember, this is about what's best for your body, so do the research you need.

138.   It is best to receive your acupuncture treatments on a regular basis. Schedule two weekly appointments for your first month and change the frequency of your appointments in function of how efficient they are. If your chronic pain or your stress is mostly gone, a monthly appointment might be enough.

139.   If your insurance policy doesn't cover acupuncture, try writing them a letter. It's important that they know that acupuncture is something that their customers want. Ask friends and family who are on the same policy to write letters as well. If you don't know what you should say, the AOMA Graduate School of Integrative Medicine has form letters available.

140.   You should find out if your acupuncturist is NCCAOM certified before you set an appointment. This national board certifies practitioners that have completed a national exam and full program. It doesn't say anything about whether their sessions are painful or not, but it does mention their educational level describing how many hours were spent in school and if they did any supervised internships at their school's clinic.

141.   Think ahead before you schedule your next acupuncture appointment. Its best that you don't have a session right before or right after you do something strenuous. If you usually workout on Wednesdays, make your appointment on a Thursday. If you're expecting to have a stressful couple of days, schedule your appointment for the following week. Acupuncture works best when you're truly able to relax.

142.   It is always best to ask a few questions to the acupuncturists you are interested in before scheduling an appointment. You need to ask if the acupuncturist is certified by the NCCAOM. The only way to get this certification is to earn a medical degree and do an acupuncture internship.

143.   To make your acupuncture benefits last longer, remember to eat before a treatment. Eating puts energy into your body, and your body will need that energy to reap all the benefits of your treatment. If you go to a session hungry, your body will utilize the stored energy it has, rather than saving that to facilitate your healing process.

144.   Inquire how long your session will last. A lot of the time your acupuncture will take about thirty minutes but it could last longer if you have a lot of health issues. Don't make any plans for the few hours following acupuncture session; this will give you relaxation time.

145.   Be sure to give yourself some extra time to get to your appointment. Rushing in at the last minute will put you into a stressful frame of mind. Stress is an inhibitor to a successful

treatment. Giving yourself a few extra minutes to arrive will allow you to calm down from the stressors of the day and let your body have the time to calm down. This calm will make your session be much more useful to you.

146.   If you are nervous about acupuncture, schedule a time to meet with a practitioner and just talk before you begin treatment. Oftentimes, you can get a lot of questions answered and some clarification about your concerns from an initial consultation. This can help to ease your mind, making your treatment process that much more effective.

147.   If acupuncture benefits are not a part of your insurance plan, start by writing the company a letter. It is possible that the company will consider amending their plan. For maximum effect, send a copy of the letter to your HR representative. Your employer may have a part in determining which benefits are included on your plan.

148.   Do not be surprised if you are a bit lightheaded our dizzy after having acupuncture done. During your session, you are laying down and blood may rush to your head. When you get up, this may cause you to feel dizzy or light

headed. Get up slowly and try to sit up for a few minutes before standing.

149.   Many people think that you have to "believe" in acupuncture in order for it to work. This is not true, however. Both children and animals, as well as adults, are treated with acupuncture, and benefit from its techniques. This makes it obvious that acupuncture is not "mystical", but a legitimate practice.

150.   Acupuncture is not an instant fix. A lot of the time you'll have to get a few different treatments. You cannot miss your sessions or you will derail your progress. If you want a relief from your pain and overall restoration of your movement, then sticking to your schedule and committing to your treatments is critical.

151.   Some patients experience a runny nose or slight flu like symptoms following an acupuncture treatment. In Chinese medicine, it is believed that colds and flus are at the root of many ailments within the body. These symptoms are just the body's way of releasing toxins, and they typically do not last for long. Do your best to keep yourself comfortable during this time, and you will soon return to optimum health.

152.   If you see red dots or bruises after an acupuncture session, don't panic! These markings aren't typical, but they aren't abnormal either, and they shouldn't be taken as a sign of a problem. It's not uncommon for people to get these after some sessions, but not others. Most markings will fade completely in a few days.

153.   The best way to locate a trustworthy acupuncturist is to ask friends, family and coworkers for a recommendation. It is likely that someone you know has used such a practitioner to help them feel great. Once you compile a list of options, you will be ready to do further research to narrow your list.

154.   You should not expect too much from your acupuncture treatments. Acupuncture can efficiently relieve pain and stress but it will not help you improve your health. You need to make some changes to your lifestyle if you suffer from chronic pain or often feel stressed. Your acupuncturist can provide you with some useful tips on how to improve your lifestyle.

155.   Don't eat too much before you go to your acupuncture session. It is important that you eat before your session to avoid dizziness and nausea, but don't overdo it. Eating too much

beforehand can cause those symptoms or worse during or after your session. Try eating a very light meal, or preferably a snack, about three hours before you get acupuncture.

156.   To protect your health, make sure that the acupuncture practitioner that you choose is certified by the health department in your state. Ask if they have been certified by the national board, completed the training program and passed any required exams. Also, find out how long they have been practicing.

157.   If you decide to follow an acupuncture treatment on the long term for a recurring problem, try scheduling your appointments ahead of time. You should meet with your acupuncturist once a week or once every other week, if possible at the same time. Continue your treatment until your problem disappears.

158.   Do not go to your acupuncture appointment hungry or full. Make sure to have a healthy snack about an hour before your appointment. Do not go with an empty stomach or after a large meal. Being to full or hungry way makes it much more difficult to relax during your acupuncture appointment.

159.   Know that acupuncture involves needles in many different areas, not just your back. Go in not being surprised if your acupuncturist needs to place needles in places like your hands, the abdomen, your scalp, or even around the ears. Remember, they know what they're doing, and this is a new style of treatment for you. Relax and let the benefits come.

160.   Often people feel extraordinarily relaxed after acupuncture. It would be wise to avoid over-stimulation by television, computers and other electronic devices for awhile afterward in order to make that relaxed feeling last. Acupuncture makes you feel good because it clears your mind. The minute you turn the television on, you will be poisoned by overload once more.

161.   You may notice your skin reacting to your treatments, possibly in the form of bruising or raised dots. These things are normal following an acupuncture session. Don't be disturbed by what you see. These marks will go away after some time and you'll feel better physically when all is said and done.

162.   When you schedule your session, mention any vitamins or supplements you've been taking.

Your acupuncturist may want you to temporarily cease taking some of them. While providing your body with extra nutrients is always a good thing, some of the supplements may cause mild side effects when taken on the day of an acupuncture session.

163.   Like with any alternative forms of medicine, it's best to keep a totally open mind in the potential benefits of acupuncture. Scientists around the globe are studying acupuncture and learning more and more about the proven benefits of it. What may seem like hog wash, can really be something pretty miraculous.

164.   Children can benefit from acupuncture too. If your child suffers from ADHD, allergies or other health ailments, sometimes acupuncture can offer answers. While not a replacement for traditional medicine, it can enhance other treatments and help to keep your child comfortable. If you decide to go this route, make sure to work with a professional who is seasoned in working with young children.

165.   Be honest with your acupuncturist. If you are experiencing pain in a certain area, they need to know about it. If you are finding the sessions frustrating because you are not seeing results,

they need to know that too. If you are not honest, you will never receive the full benefits of your treatments or find the relief you are hoping for.

166.   Certain folks undergo emotional releases while being treated with acupuncture. This should not come as a surprise. You shouldn't be ashamed to show your acupuncturist your feelings because this person is used to patients displaying emotions during treatment. This release shows the treatment is actually effective.

167.   It is important not to have an acupuncture treatment on an empty stomach. This can increase the possibility of certain side-effects, such as dizziness and nausea. Instead, eat a light meal before your appointment. Avoid any foods that could cause nausea, including fried, or overly greasy foods that could upset your stomach.

168.   Always consider your comfort level when you meet an acupuncturist. Are you going to be comfortable with this person when you are laying on a table without clothes? Will you feel okay when he is putting needles in various parts of your body? Do you trust him? If you answered no, it is time to look elsewhere for a different practitioner.

169.   During your consultation with your acupuncturist, it is likely that you will have to show him your tongue at some point. Taking the pulse of the tongue is a way for them to see how the energy in your body is flowing. He may also check your blood pressure, heart rate, temperature, and talk to you about your level of stress. All of this data helps build your treatment plan.

170.   It is best to receive your acupuncture treatments on a regular basis. Schedule two weekly appointments for your first month and change the frequency of your appointments in function of how efficient they are. If your chronic pain or your stress is mostly gone, a monthly appointment might be enough.

171.   It is important to relax before going to an acupuncture treatment. If you are tense, the needles will not be able to get past your clenched muscles. Breathing deeply just before the treatment or listening to some relaxing music should help. If you are having problems with tensed muscles, let your acupuncturist know about this problem.

172.   It is important to let your acupuncturist know about the vitamins or medications you are taking before the beginning of your treatment. Some pills can affect your system and counteract the effects of an acupuncture session. You might have to stop taking your medication or vitamins for a while if you want to get good results from acupuncture.

173.   You need to wait a while if you want acupuncture to work. The true impact of acupuncture may not appear until multiple sessions have occurred. Don't be disappointed if you do not feel the full effect after a single session. For this reason, you should follow your treatment plan and be patient to allow acupuncture to work.

174.   Acupuncture produces different effects in different people. Some people report that they feel extremely relaxed after a session, while others notice a burst of extra energy. A common benefit reported by most patients is an overall sense of well-being and fitness. These feelings are in addition to achieving the pain relief they were seeking.

175.   Be choosy when scheduling your treatments. Don't make an appointment too close to when

you will be doing strenuous activity. You should never schedule a session in the middle to two other activities, as your stress level is likely to be elevated. This may make it difficult for you to relax.

176.   If you are pregnant, past your due date and wanting to get labor started, consider using acupuncture. This pain-free, natural practice can pinpoint specific parts of the body which can bring on contractions and help labor to progress. It is important to only use this past your due date however, so as to avoid pre-term labor which might be dangerous to the baby's health.

177.   Avoid alcohol in the days before your session. Acupuncture is intended to clear the body and mind. The use of alcohol contraindicates the benefits of acupuncture. If you drank a lot the previous night and still feel a hangover, you should probably reschedule your appointment so you can obtain the maximum benefits.

178.   Talk to your acupuncturist about their hours and determine how long you will be there for an appointment. This information can help you figure out what part of the day would be best for you to set something up. Ideally, you want to

head in for a treatment when you are fairly relaxed, as you will get the best results that way.

179.   If you suffer with frequent migraine headaches and have yet to find relief, think about visiting a local acupuncture practice. Often times migraines are caused or exacerbated by stress and physical tension building up in your back and neck muscles. The acupuncture professional you visit should be able to alleviate some of this tension, providing you with some much needed relief.

180.   Acupuncture is relatively painless. You should experience little to no pain during an acupuncture session. The needles are very tiny. Although you may feel a slight sensation to inform you that the needle is inside your body, it will not hurt.

181.   It is always important that you feel comfortable with the person preforming acupuncture on you. Being uncomfortable and remaining tense through the treatments can end up being counterproductive to your therapy. Find an acupuncturist that you feel totally comfortable with and once you do, stick with that person. You can even give other people referrals.

182.   A search of the Internet may yield good results when you are seeking an acupuncturist. You can type in your zip, state, city and "acupuncturist" into some search engine and look at the results. AcuFinder.com and NCCAOM.org also provide search engines you can use. NCCAOM will be the agency that licenses acupuncturists in the United states which will assist you in finding practitioners that are licensed in your area.

183.   If you want to get the most out of your acupuncture sessions, take steps to improve your diet. Eat more whole foods, and do your best to eliminate processed sugar. Replace coffee with tea, and drink plenty of water. Acupuncture releases toxins, and bad foods will only bring them back.

184.   Receiving acupuncture treatments regularly will eventually help you become more aware of your body. You might feel uncomfortable and even experience pains that you never noticed before. This is a negative side effect but it is also a sign that your acupuncture treatment is working. Explore acupuncture further to correct the new problems you are noticing.

185.   If acupuncture benefits are not a part of your insurance plan, start by writing the company a letter. It is possible that the company will consider amending their plan. For maximum effect, send a copy of the letter to your HR representative. Your employer may have a part in determining which benefits are included on your plan.

186.   Some patients experience a runny nose or slight flu like symptoms following an acupuncture treatment. In Chinese medicine, it is believed that colds and flus are at the root of many ailments within the body. These symptoms are just the body's way of releasing toxins, and they typically do not last for long. Do your best to keep yourself comfortable during this time, and you will soon return to optimum health.

187.   Before going to an acupuncture session, eat something light. If your too full, your results might not be optimal. Do not go in for a treatment when you are feeling hungry either. If you go in for treatment when you are hungry, you may experience unwelcome nausea or dizziness.

188.   There is really nothing to be scared of when it comes to acupuncture. The needles that are

used do not cause pain and are usually very thin. Pain will not be an issue.

189.   Some people find acupuncture treatments are quite effective for migraine headaches. One very positive aspect of this type of alternative treatment is the lack of any side effects. Even though very fine needles are inserted into the flesh at specific points, most people do not feel any pain at all from the procedure.

190.   If you have some fear of acupuncture because you think that it is going to hurt, ask your acupuncturist about techniques in painless needling. Ask questions about where he learned that technique and how long he has been practicing it. Only go with practitioners who have had multiple years of experience.

191.   For the best experience at your acupuncture treatment, wear comfortable clothing. This will allow the acupuncturist to access any pressure points that are important for your treatment. Also, it is a good idea to write down your symptoms and bring a list of problem areas so that you can give specific details for him to target.

192.   If you are skeptical about acupuncture, don't move forward with it until you've alleviated whatever is holding you back. Acupuncture is not an area that everyone is immediately comfortable with. It involves needles for one, and the mindset is quite different than Westerners are used to. Learn all that you can prior, and make a conscious decision once you're confident in it.

193.   Avoid having coffee before your treatment. You should abstain for about two hours before an appointment. This restriction is due to the fact that coffee is a stimulant which works in direct opposition to the goals of your acupuncture session. Coffee also makes the acupuncturist's job more difficult because it is harder to get accurate heart rate readings.

194.   Know what you're getting into. Acupuncture involves dealing with tiny needles. There is no way to get around that, so come to terms with it before you arrive for your first appointment. As an acupuncturist if they have any times for feeling more comfortable with needles, so you don't have to worry.

195.   Acupuncture pins are meant to target the chi in the body. Chi refers to your life force energy.

There is an energy channel in the body and anytime there is an obstruction or anything that interferes with it, it takes the form of a physical issue in the body like pain. The pins in acupuncture can help redirect or balance the chi in your body.

196.   Make sure you ask if your health insurance covers your acupuncture appointments. Acupuncture is often costly, particularly when multiple sessions are needed. You may want to change your insurance policy or look for a new provider if you decide that long-term acupuncture treatment is right for you and you want to get it covered.

197.   Use a little visualization to help your acupuncture treatment along. Visualize the pain or injury escaping as the needle is put in place, and focus on a feeling of numbness around the insertion site to help yourself to avoid discomfort. Visualization is a very powerful thing, and it can make your treatments more effective and long lasting.

198.   If you're feeling a little sore after an acupuncture session, the best way to treat that soreness is with heat. Post-session pain is usually caused by blockages, and ice may only exacerbate

the problem. Most soreness is gone within 24 hours, so a hot bath and a good night's sleep should do the trick.

199.　It is always important that you feel comfortable with the person preforming acupuncture on you. Being uncomfortable and remaining tense through the treatments can end up being counterproductive to your therapy. Find an acupuncturist that you feel totally comfortable with and once you do, stick with that person. You can even give other people referrals.

200.　If you feel very tired after an acupuncture treatment, you should get some rest. Acupuncture is supposed to give you some energy but you will not get this positive effect if you need some sleep. It is important to get eight hours of sleep a night until your next treatment.

201.　Do not be surprised if you are a bit lightheaded our dizzy after having acupuncture done. During your session, you are laying down and blood may rush to your head. When you get up, this may cause you to feel dizzy or light headed. Get up slowly and try to sit up for a few minutes before standing.

202.   If you are really tense about acupuncture, consider looking for a practitioner that offers "community" sessions. These are acupuncture sessions where multiple people are in a room receiving treatments. Some people find this community aspect very relaxing. Don't worry: Any consultation is done in private before the sessions, so medical histories are not shared among the group.

203.   Be honest with your acupuncturist. If you are experiencing pain in a certain area, they need to know about it. If you are finding the sessions frustrating because you are not seeing results, they need to know that too. If you are not honest, you will never receive the full benefits of your treatments or find the relief you are hoping for.

204.   It is important to relax before going to an acupuncture treatment. If you are tense, the needles will not be able to get past your clenched muscles. Breathing deeply just before the treatment or listening to some relaxing music should help. If you are having problems with tensed muscles, let your acupuncturist know about this problem.

205. Do you suffer from chronic pain, but are leery about taking prescription medication to help it? If so, then acupuncture might be for you! Acupuncture targets pressure points in the body to relieve pain and stress. This medical practice is used all over the world and is a great alternative to prescription medications.

206. If you'd like to get more out of your acupuncture sessions, start cleansing. A good cleanse will free your body of toxins, which means acupuncture will be more effective. During this time, you may also want to detox from substances like alcohol. Ask your acupuncturist to recommend a good detox diet.

207. After an acupuncture session, remember to hydrate yourself properly. A good rule of thumb is to consume at least six glasses of water following a session. Acupuncture can cause you to release toxins from the body, and you need to drink water to flush those toxins from your system.

208. If you often feel sluggish and like you're running out of gas long before the end of your day, consider what acupuncture may be able to do for you. Most people are under the impression that it's just for pain, but that isn't the

whole truth! Acupuncture can help rejuvenate you and give you more energy to deal with your day.

209.   Consider bringing your own pillow to an acupuncture session. You want to make yourself as comfortable as possible during the hour or so that it takes to place the needles, and sometimes having a little comfort at home can help. Alternately, a comfortable throw or a favorite pair of slippers might offer you just the comfort you are looking for.

210.   If acupuncture benefits are not a part of your insurance plan, start by writing the company a letter. It is possible that the company will consider amending their plan. For maximum effect, send a copy of the letter to your HR representative. Your employer may have a part in determining which benefits are included on your plan.

211.   When you schedule your session, mention any vitamins or supplements you've been taking. Your acupuncturist may want you to temporarily cease taking some of them. While providing your body with extra nutrients is always a good thing, some of the supplements may cause mild side

effects when taken on the day of an acupuncture session.

212.   Acupuncture can sometimes cause you to experience emotional release. Many people experience a variety of emotions during their treatment. The acupuncturist sees emotions such as people crying or laughing over nothing. Emotional release should be seen as a sign that you're getting the full benefits of the treatment.

213.   Once you finish a treatment, do not head right to the gym. While some exercise is okay, it should not be anything too intensive. For instance, if you generally run a mile each evening after work, scale it back to a walk instead. Continue to live your life as you normally with, just add in a few modifications.

214.   Once you finish up with the acupuncturist, stay away from both coffee and alcohol. These drinks dehydrate you, and that is bad for your treatment. Acupuncture can cause the release of toxins, which have to be flushed out of your system. Alcohol and coffee will inhibit that process, so they should be avoided.

215.   Acupuncture is not an instant fix. In many cases, multiple treatments are necessary. Do not

miss any of your sessions if you want the best results. You must commit to all of the sessions to see true relief form your pain.

216.   You might be more sensitive than usual after an acupuncture treatment. Do not worry if you experience mood swings or seem to cry very easily. This is a sign that your acupuncture treatment is working well. These symptoms should eventually disappear as you get used to receiving acupuncture treatments regularly.

217.   Feeling a need to urinate frequently after an acupuncture session is normal. This is one of the many ways that the body releases toxins, and it can also help with bloating and water retention within the body. Acupuncture helps with all of these things, thus the need for frequent urination. Continue to drink water as normal until the symptoms subside.

218.   You may feel very tired after an acupuncture session. This isn't common, but it does happen. If you experience fatigue, there is no reason to worry. Simply do your best to rest throughout the day and head to bed an hour or so before you usually do. You should feel great when you wake up.

219.   Study up on acupuncture. You've probably heard of it, and if you have, you know it involves needles. But there is much more to acupuncture, and you should get a better picture of it prior to making any decisions about it. Remember, this is about what's best for your body, so do the research you need.

220.   Bring along something to comfort yourself. Particularly for your first session in acupuncture, bring a comfortable blanket or pillow to ease your tension. This can reduce the stress and put you in a place to better accept treatment. Ask your acupuncturist to make sure you can bring a familiar object with you.

221.   The benefits of acupuncture often take a while to see. It takes a while for results to begin to be felt. Be patient and pay attention to how you are feeling. Thus, give it time for acupuncture to work on your body.

222.   Keep in mind that it may take some time for you to feel the full benefits from your acupuncture treatments. It may take more than one or two visits to find relief from pain or improvement in your conditions. Make sure you are ready to commit to the full program recommended.

223.   Falling asleep during an acupuncture treatment is not uncommon. You should not feel like the treatment was wasted because you feel asleep. Going to sleep during a treatment is actually a sign that you are able to fully relax and experience a sensation known as Qi. You will probably notice that your pain or stress is gone when you wake up.

224.   Do not drink alcohol before your appointment. Such chemicals will inhibit your ability to relax and clear your mind. Alcohol can impede the goal of getting rid of the cobwebs. If you have a hangover, you may just want to reschedule the session so that you do not miss out on all of the benefits.

225.   To protect your health, make sure that the acupuncture practitioner that you choose is certified by the health department in your state. Ask if they have been certified by the national board, completed the training program and passed any required exams. Also, find out how long they have been practicing.

226.   Talk to your acupuncturist about their hours and determine how long you will be there for an appointment. This information can help you

figure out what part of the day would be best for you to set something up. Ideally, you want to head in for a treatment when you are fairly relaxed, as you will get the best results that way.

227.   If you feel pain during an acupuncture session, let your practitioner know. A small prick is normal when the needle is inserted, but you should not feel anything beyond that. More intense pain can mean that the practitioner hit a nerve, and this can cause you to experience adverse side effects if it is not immediately addressed.

228.   Chronic pains can be cured with acupuncture. If you often experience pain in your lower back or in your joints, you should find a good acupuncturist. You should notice a difference after your first treatment but additional sessions will be needed to make sure your chronic pain does not come back.

229.   Acupuncture is not limited to use on humans. Many veterinarians are starting to offer this service, and it is benefiting dogs and cats alike. When issues such as arthritis or bone deterioration are present, acupuncture can ease a pet's suffering and sometimes prolong their life.

Ask about this if your pet is showing signs of concern.

230.   When you schedule your session, mention any vitamins or supplements you've been taking. Your acupuncturist may want you to temporarily cease taking some of them. While providing your body with extra nutrients is always a good thing, some of the supplements may cause mild side effects when taken on the day of an acupuncture session.

231.   While acupuncture has been proven to be a very safe technique, some people have been known to suffer from mild side-effects. Some of these side-effects include: lightheadedness, nausea or fainting. These conditions are quite rare. However, it is important to discuss possible side-effects with the practitioner before having any procedure done.

232.   Listen to music during your acupuncture session. Choose something that relaxes you completely, not something that well rev you up. Remember, it's all about relaxing. Classical music is a great choice, or you could opt for a relaxing form of jazz. It's ok if you're relaxed to the point of near sleep. That will help your muscles respond to the treatment.

233.   Inquire about the experience of an acupuncturist before you allow a treatment to be done. This is especially important if you are getting acupuncture done at a place that has more than one acupuncturist. Make sure that they have some kind of credentials and experience with the process, so you can be confident about the work they're going to do.

234.   Get a full consultation before accepting any treatment. Acupuncture is all about full body well-being, and there are many techniques that differ based off of the issues at hand. A professional practitioner will never give a treatment without first having a serious consultation in regard to your current health and overall mood. It'll change how they go about treating you.

235.   It is important not to have an acupuncture treatment on an empty stomach. This can increase the possibility of certain side-effects, such as dizziness and nausea. Instead, eat a light meal before your appointment. Avoid any foods that could cause nausea, including fried, or overly greasy foods that could upset your stomach.

236.   As you choose an acupuncturist, research is key. Sadly, not every practitioner available to you will be the best choice. Start with a list of recommendations and contact each. Ask for references and follow up on them. Check out the cleanliness of their office and ask about their needle cleaning practices.

237.   When deciding which acupuncturist to select, you should consider their education. Medical professionals who can give you acupuncture include chiropractors, acupuncturists, and doctors trained to practice acupuncture. The choice is up to you and your preferences, but it is essential to know what kind of training your acupuncturist has had.

238.   Do not be intimidated by needles! That being said, many will be intimidated. It is common to feel this way; however, acupuncture has been around for centuries. Millions have had this procedure done and are better off for it. Grab your fear, toss it aside and make the appointment. You will be happy that you did.

239.   Determine if and how your insurance plan covers acupuncture. Some plans cover acupuncture only if you are referred by your regular practitioner for a medical condition.

Other plans cover acupuncture visits as wellness visits. Find out if your health insurance covers acupuncture so you can save some cash on the procedure.

240. When beginning acupuncture treatments, you should keep participating until you have received a full round. Never stop halfway, as this will not allow you to see the full benefit. Even though you feel great, you may not have immediate results. Finish the treatments to see how great you can really feel.

241. Schedule a consultation before choosing a acupuncturist. The acupuncture technician should inquire about the type of pain you're experiencing. Let them know everything that is going on. Inform them of how your pain is affecting your daily life. Every bit you tell your acupuncturist will help them to help you.

242. Take it easy on yourself following your treatment. Chose activities post session that will be non stressful and relaxing. The benefits of acupuncture continue on well after your treatment is over. If you put yourself under stress immediately afterwards you will be taking away some of the benefits of your treatment.

243.   If you often feel sluggish and like you're running out of gas long before the end of your day, consider what acupuncture may be able to do for you. Most people are under the impression that it's just for pain, but that isn't the whole truth! Acupuncture can help rejuvenate you and give you more energy to deal with your day.

244.   Chronic pains can be cured with acupuncture. If you often experience pain in your lower back or in your joints, you should find a good acupuncturist. You should notice a difference after your first treatment but additional sessions will be needed to make sure your chronic pain does not come back.

245.   Recent studies show that acupuncture can help those on medication for depression and anxiety. For starters, patients are able to reduce their dosage of medication when they also have acupuncture because the procedure reduces feelings of nervousness and sadness. Acupuncture also reduces the side effects of depression medications, like weight gain and nausea.

246.   If your health insurance plan doesn't cover acupuncture, start writing letters. If you have

colleagues who wish to undergo acupuncture treatment, recruit them to speak to Human Resources officers. You may find that the insurance company will respond well and add it to the insurance plan if enough people are interested.

247.   Acupuncture is recognized as an effective treatment for a lot of different ailments and diseases by the medical world. If you are considering having this type of treatment, you might want to check with your insurance company first. Many insurance companies will actually cover the cost of acupuncture treatments.

248.   Do not be surprised if you are a bit lightheaded our dizzy after having acupuncture done. During your session, you are laying down and blood may rush to your head. When you get up, this may cause you to feel dizzy or light headed. Get up slowly and try to sit up for a few minutes before standing.

249.   If you are looking for an acupuncturist near you, try asking around for recommendations. You can ask friends, family, coworkers, etc. If any of them get acupuncture treatments or have in the past, try asking them who did it, what it

was like and if they would recommend them to you. It is usually better to get acupuncturist referrals from people you trust than calling about someone in a printed ad.

250.   Verify the length of your appointment when you set it up. You have to keep yourself relaxed when you get through with an appointment and it can be stressful if you have a bunch of things planned for later in the day. See how long it'll take and schedule accordingly.

251.   Once you finish up with the acupuncturist, stay away from both coffee and alcohol. These drinks dehydrate you, and that is bad for your treatment. Acupuncture can cause the release of toxins, which have to be flushed out of your system. Alcohol and coffee will inhibit that process, so they should be avoided.

252.   You should not drink coffee before an acupuncture treatment. Coffee has stimulation properties and will make it hard for you to relax during your treatment. Your acupuncturist will have a hard time measuring your pulse if you drink coffee. If possible, wait until after your appointment to have some coffee.

253.   Feeling a need to urinate frequently after an acupuncture session is normal. This is one of the many ways that the body releases toxins, and it can also help with bloating and water retention within the body. Acupuncture helps with all of these things, thus the need for frequent urination. Continue to drink water as normal until the symptoms subside.

254.   Keep a journal about your sessions. Record your feelings as well as any changes you feel after each treatment. Then you'll be able to show what you've written to the acupuncturist. This will allow them to check up on if they need to adjust of modify the treatment you've been getting.

255.   Be certain to allow plenty of time for your acupuncture treatments to take effect. The full health benefit of acupuncture may only become apparent after several sessions. It may take more than one session to feel the full effect. So, be patient, go to each session, and give it time to be effective.

256.   Never allow an acupuncturist to use the needles he or she uses on other patients. If the needles he or she is about to use on you don't come from a brand new sealed package, be sure to ask where they did come from. A professional

doctor never reuses needles. If they do, this is a clear warning that you should move on to someone else.

257.	Some people find acupuncture treatments are quite effective for migraine headaches. One very positive aspect of this type of alternative treatment is the lack of any side effects. Even though very fine needles are inserted into the flesh at specific points, most people do not feel any pain at all from the procedure.

258.	Ask your acupuncturist about their education. Acupuncturists need to go to medical school for four years before completing an internship. The internship should last at least eighteen months. If your acupuncturist cannot prove they have this kind of educational background, you should find another specialized doctor who can treat you.

259.	Make sure the acupuncturist you go to performs painless acupuncture. Painless treatments are very popular in the U.S. but pain can actually play a part in relieving your stress or treating your health problem. You should not try these treatments until you know more about acupuncture and are ready to try a more advanced treatment.

260.   You should drink plenty of water before you attend your scheduled acupuncture session. It has been shown that people who are well hydrated respond better to treatments. While you should not consume a lot of food before a session, it is a great idea for you to drink a good amount of water.

261.   Finish your entire treatment plan before making a decision on its efficacy for you It is never a good idea to give up on treatments before you finish the complete cycle. You may feel better by the end of your session; however, the results may not be complete. Allow the prescribed treatment length to run its course and then you can determine how your body has coped with it all.

262.   Talk to your acupuncturist about their hours and determine how long you will be there for an appointment. This information can help you figure out what part of the day would be best for you to set something up. Ideally, you want to head in for a treatment when you are fairly relaxed, as you will get the best results that way.

263.   Acupuncture is based on the Chinese theory that stimulating specific nerve centers can relieve

pain and some diseases. Very fine needles are inserted at these points and manipulated either manually or by electricity. The alternative practice of acupressure is sometimes as effective as acupuncture, but its success often depends of the type of ailment needing treatment.

264.   Know what you're getting into. Acupuncture involves dealing with tiny needles. There is no way to get around that, so come to terms with it before you arrive for your first appointment. As an acupuncturist if they have any times for feeling more comfortable with needles, so you don't have to worry.

265.   The first time you have an acupuncture session, you should watch out for fatigue. Some people get a burst of energy after an appointment, but others feel physically drained. Make sure you don't have anything important scheduled after your appointment so that you can get rest if you need it.

266.   Herbal treatments could be suggested to you by your acupuncturist before treatment. Be warned that even herbs can interact poorly with your prescription drugs. Do not mix any herbal substances with other medications without prior approval from your physician.

267.   While visiting your acupuncturist is a huge part of the healing process, he will likely send you home with some things to do at home. These self-care treatments may include pressing on pressure points or even relaxation techniques to help reduce stress. Always do your homework to speed up recovery!

268.   Get yourself into a relaxed state before beginning your acupuncture treatment. Life is full of tensions, from work assignments to family arguments. Leave those behind when you get on the acupuncture table. The more you're able to relax, the better you'll respond to the treatments given. That's where you want to be.

269.   Acupuncture is known to help problems with digestion. Some treatments can help with the natural cycles of the body like digestion. Speak to your practitioner about what you eat in order to bolster your results. Keep going until your digestion is back to normal.

270.   Stress isn't the only problem you will notice a reduction in over time: pain will also begin to lessen after each treatment. Pains may be as severe as menstrual pains or carpal tunnel, yet these thin needles will be enough to encourage a

positive response from the body. Migraines and other similar conditions are also treatable through acupuncture.

271.   Wear loose clothing when going for an acupuncture appointment. You want to be as comfortable as possible while you are having your procedure. Wear clothes similar to what you would wear in your home.

272.   Before you go to your appointment, learn more about acupuncture. No one likes needles, but they are necessary in this type of treatment. That's just a part of it. If they make you nervous, you can get over it by facing that fear head on. If you have to, find others who have had acupuncture and can tell you how their experience was, so you don't worry.

273.   If you are nervous about acupuncture, and you are not sure if it is right for you, do not be afraid to ask questions. Believe it or not, one of the most common inquiries is whether or not the acupuncturist practices a painless style of treatment. Your fears may be eased when you hear some of the answers.

274.   After an acupuncture treatment, you may feel tremendous energy. A lot of clients have had

a boost of energy for quite some time after having an acupuncture session. People are usually relaxed immediately after a treatment, but the energy boost soon follows.

275.   It is always best to ask a few questions to the acupuncturists you are interested in before scheduling an appointment. You need to ask if the acupuncturist is certified by the NCCAOM. The only way to get this certification is to earn a medical degree and do an acupuncture internship.

276.   Acupuncture is not a good option if you feel very stressed. Do not hesitate to cancel a treatment if you had an extremely stressful day. Acupuncture will not be very efficient if your muscles are tense and the toxins released during the treatment could actually make your stress even worse.

277.   Inquire whether you should do anything before or after your treatment. Your acupuncturist may want you to take certain actions, such as laying down for a while after the treatment, or drinking a full glass of water. Find out before your treatment, so you know what to expect each time.

278.   Did you know that acupuncture can be of assistance to those looking to quit smoking? The actual acupuncture procedure helps people deal with the side effects of nicotine addiction, like irritability, cravings and jitters. It calms the patient down so they are better able to deal with these side effects.

279.   Avoid drinking alcohol for at least several days after having acupuncture treatments. When you have this type of procedure done, it releases a lot of toxins into your body. These toxins sometimes cause the body to become dehydrated, and having alcohol in your system will only make the situation worse.

280.   Like with any alternative forms of medicine, it's best to keep a totally open mind in the potential benefits of acupuncture. Scientists around the globe are studying acupuncture and learning more and more about the proven benefits of it. What may seem like hog wash, can really be something pretty miraculous.

281.   Before going to your acupuncture session, have a light snack. Do not overeat or go in with an empty stomach. This will help prevent dizziness or feeling nauseous. You want to be relaxed and comfortable. If you are hungry or

bloated, you will not be relaxed and could hinder your treatment.

282.   It is not uncommon to experience muscle twitching during an acupuncture treatment. You should not worry about muscle twitching but let your acupuncturist know if you experience a muscle spasm. This can easily be treated in a few minutes at the end of your appointment. If you repeatedly get this problem, try a different treatment.

283.   You may feel very tired after an acupuncture session. This isn't common, but it does happen. If you experience fatigue, there is no reason to worry. Simply do your best to rest throughout the day and head to bed an hour or so before you usually do. You should feel great when you wake up.

284.   Sometimes acupuncture can leave you feeling sore, particularly on your feet and hands. Generally, the soreness will go away in a day's time, although you may experience some issues for up to a week later. Simply try to stay off your feet as much as possible, and allow your hands to rest as well.

285.   The best way to locate a trustworthy acupuncturist is to ask friends, family and coworkers for a recommendation. It is likely that someone you know has used such a practitioner to help them feel great. Once you compile a list of options, you will be ready to do further research to narrow your list.

286.   When you have a chronic condition, an acupuncturist will recommend daily treatments for a month to see good results. Sadly, most of us can't afford to see them that frequently, so two or three sessions a week will be the maximum. In that case, results will still appear, but it will take longer.

287.   While it may be easy to ask your chosen practitioner questions about the care they give, if you don't know the answer you are looking for, it will be no help at all! Learn about how a good acupuncturist diagnoses your condition and then ask the question expecting the answer you have researched.

288.   Make sure you schedule your acupuncture appointment at a point in the day that is relatively calm for you. For instance, if you know you have a big work presentation, don't set up your appointment for right before or right after

that, as you will likely be stressed out for your treatment.

Make sure you are breathing deep during an acupuncture session. If you tend to hold your breathe when you are tense, you may be doing yourself a big disservice during treatment. Take big breathes, and let your muscles fully relax. They'll then be ready to accept the needles and other methods used in the sessions.

www.ingramcontent.com/pod-product-compliance
Lightning Source LLC
Chambersburg PA
CBHW060753260726
48660CB00002B/596